Healing /
Anal Fissuᵣₑ

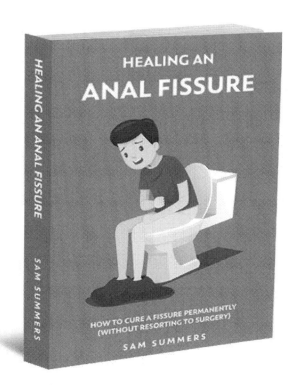

Healing An Anal Fissure:
How To Cure A Fissure Permanently
(Without Resorting To Surgery)

Sam Summers

Read This First

Thank you for purchasing Healing An Anal Fissure

You will get the most value from this book if you download the Audio Book, the Cheat Sheets and subscribe to the 30 days of email support.

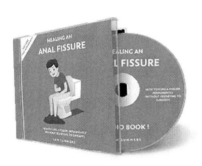 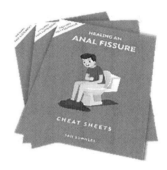

1. Read this book: Healing An Anal Fissure

2. Listen to the accompanying Audio Book and download the Cheat Sheets:

https://www.HealAnalFissure.com/get-audio-book

3. Subscribe to the 30 Days of Email Support:

https://www.HealAnalFissure.com/support

Copyright Notice

Healing An Anal Fissure: How To Cure A Fissure Permanently (Without Resorting To Surgery)

© SAM SUMMERS

Heal Anal Fissure, https://www.healanalfissure.com

Legal Notice

The purpose of this book is to educate and guide and the advice herein may not be suitable for your own situation.

The author recommends that you carry out your own due diligence.

Any brand names or product names mentioned are trademarks or registered trademarks of their respective companies.

Disclaimer

You should assume that the author has an affiliate relationship with the products that are recommended inside of this book and will receive compensation for purchases made through the referral links.

The author intends to collect revenue generated from product referrals and use it for marketing costs to help this book reach more sufferers of this unfortunate condition.

In the present Internet age, reaching a large audience through effective marketing usually involves significant resources and up-front expenditure.

There is no obligation for you to buy any of the products that the author recommends. Nor are you obliged to use the author's affiliate links.

You may choose to carry out a quick search in a search engine and find the recommended products through your own efforts.

If you do make a purchase through the referral links (at no extra cost to yourself), the author thanks you for your trust and for helping this information to reach others that are suffering from an anal fissure.

Note: links to all of the recommended products in this book can be found at: https://www.healanalfissure.com/products

Dedication

This book is dedicated to anyone that is currently suffering from, or has experienced, an anal fissure.

I understand what you are going through and I would implore you: please do not give up hope.

This condition is far more common than you realize even though it's not talked about much.

Anal fissures do not discriminate on age or status and can affect anyone from any background.

But many people are embarrassed to open up emotionally and get the support they need from their Physician and from their family and friends.

Please read this book in full and then go back and take action on all of the advice that I've given.

A single treatment on its own may not be enough to heal you. But combining several treatments is more powerful and can put you on the road to recovery.

As you start to heal you will notice an improvement with your bowel movements.

*** If you are in immediate pain and need treatment fast, please skip the following sections and jump straight to chapters 6 & 7 where I cover pain relief and treatments for your fissure ***

If you follow all the recommendations in chapters 6 & 7 you will improve your chances of being able to avoid surgery.

You can then come back and read the other chapters once your pain is under control.

I have structured this book specifically to give you what you need - i.e. something actionable.

The information in this book has enabled many others to heal their fissure.

I was able to recover and I believe that you can also recover, using the methods in this book, if you follow the advice and keep a positive mindset.

If you have questions about healing your fissure and would like to receive personal support, via a 1-1 consultation, you can arrange a session directly with the author.

Visit: https://www.healanalfissure.com/consultation

Note: The author reserves the right to remove 1-1 support at any time based on demand and his availability.

If you are considering a 1-1 support session, the author recommends that you schedule an appointment **now** by visiting the URL above.

Table of Contents

A Note To The Reader

The time that it takes to heal a fissure will vary from person to person.

There are many factors to consider, for example:

- The length/depth of your fissure
- How long you've had the fissure
- Your diet
- Body weight
- Stress
- Exercise
- The state of your health

Each of these factors will have a bearing on the time that it takes for you to heal.

Some people can heal within days whilst for others (particularly if your fissure is chronic, i.e. you've had it for longer than 6 weeks) it may take months to heal.

The time that it takes for the elasticity of the skin in the anal area to return back to normal, after a fissure is healed, can be as long as 2 years.

My aim is to help you cure your anal fissure quickly and naturally without having to spend thousands of dollars on surgery.

We all have different bodies and it's possible that some of the recommended products in this book may not suit you.

Keep a positive attitude: the products that I've recommended have worked for me and many others. Each of us managed to cure our fissure without resorting to surgery.

Some products will provide more relief than others but there's no way of knowing which ones work until you try.

Using all the recommended products in this book will give you a better opportunity to heal naturally.

There may be a small number of people for whom surgery is the only realistic option. If this is you, I recommend carefully researching the right Colorectal Surgeon (CRS).

For more information on finding a CRS, read chapter 12.

A study in the Nursing2008 journal found that surgery for anal fissures carries a risk of permanent injury to the anal sphincter, leading to fecal incontinence in 30% of patients:

https://tinyurl.com/lww-2008

Full URL:
https://journals.lww.com/nursing/fulltext/2008/08000/anal_fissure__how_to_support_spontaneous_healing.50.aspx

I pray for your success in your path back to normal, pain free bowel movements.

Chapter 1

Personal Information About The Author

I am a regular guy, just like you or someone else in your family. I'm now in my 40's. I'm married and have 2 children that are in school.

Turning 40 was a real wake up call for me. It was almost like an invisible force had flicked a switch in my body.

My metabolism felt like it slowed down overnight.

Every year, my family and I try to go on vacation during the summer holidays when the kids are off from school. In previous years, I'd start slimming down about 3 months before the holiday to try and get a respectable looking 'beach body'.

I didn't want to be known as "fat dad".

Slimming down usually involved cutting out the junk (takeaways and desserts) and hitting the treadmill 2-3 times a week.

Until my late 30's, this method worked for me and I'd typically drop 7-10 pounds in weight and look respectable by the holiday.

(Of course, I'd indulge during the holiday and after returning back home and so the weight would creep back on within a few weeks.)

Struggles With My Weight

After I turned 40 however, things changed.

I was doing the same things as I'd done in previous years but this time the weight didn't just drop off. Maybe you can relate?

By the time we left for our summer holiday, I'd only lost 1 pound. There were other changes too. My energy levels had dropped. I felt less 'fit' than I had in previous years.

Recovery times from any type of exercise were taking longer. I felt tired and grumpy more quickly than usual.

In desperation I hit the gym.

I'd read in a men's magazine that from our mid 30's, men begin to lose muscle mass and this trend becomes more noticeable aged 40 onwards.

I figured that if I could start weight training again, I'd be able to improve my physique and lose some of the stubborn pounds around my belly that were giving me a "dad body".

Changing my diet and upgrading my exercise regime worked but it took time and consistency.

Since turning 40, I have exercised consistently every week. Instead of driving my kids to school, we now go by walk. I also go to the gym 1-2 times a week.

My weight is now back in the normal range (according to my BMI - Body Mass Index).

Fissures Don't Discriminate

The reason I'm sharing my weight problems with you is because even though I now lead a healthy lifestyle, I still got an anal fissure.

So, if it can happen to a healthy person, it can happen to anyone.

Medical advice says that most people suffer from fissures between the ages of 15-40.

I've been vegetarian for several years now. I drink plenty of water and have enough fiber in my diet.

How I Got A Fissure

I'm not 100% sure why I got an anal fissure but I suspect there were 2 reasons for it:

1) Over consumption of nuts: I'm addicted to all of them, especially the salted and roasted ones, and probably wasn't chewing them enough.

2) Bad exercise habits in the gym: weight training, especially in the lower body, can pull your muscles and cause tears.

As we age, the elasticity in our muscles deteriorates and this can cause all kinds of mobility issues in our joints and ligaments.

Experiencing Anal Fissure Pain

The pain from an anal fissure is the worst pain that I have ever experienced. You probably feel the same.

A few years ago, I had my wisdom teeth taken out because my dentist told me that I had overcrowding in my mouth.

One side of my wisdom teeth did not come out cleanly and the dentist had to wiggle the tooth to pull it out. This caused excruciating nerve pain and I suffered for days afterwards.

Looking back, I can say that the pain from having a wisdom tooth out paled into comparison from the pain of having an anal fissure.

There are hundreds of nerve endings in the anus. At its worst, I was left in tears during (and shortly after) a bowel movement. I used to dread going to the bathroom because I knew the pain that was coming after.

As humans we are programmed to avoid pain but with bowel movements there is no avoidance. Sure, you can delay a movement but that just makes it worse when you do go.

The harsh reality is we have to eat in order to survive. And what we put into our mouths eventually comes out through our bowel movements.

In desperation, I even tried a 48 hour fast. It felt great not having a bowel movement on the second day of the fast and I was able to temporarily control the pain using medication.

But inevitably I had to eat. Experiencing hunger pangs and fading energy levels is no fun.

And with family responsibilities towards my wife and 2 kids, I knew that I had to eat to keep going. There was no escape... I had to get on with life.

Avoiding food, and the inevitable bowel movement the next day, was not a solution even though at times I wish it was.

Until you experience the pain from an anal fissure, I don't think it's possible to understand what it feels like.

There were days when I couldn't do anything productive.

I was literally rolling around in bed, desperately massaging my anus and waiting for the painkillers to kick in to give me some temporary relief from the agony.

I'm opening up here to let you know that I understand exactly what you're going through. The pain is so strong that at times it can make you feel suicidal.

Out of sheer desperation to avoid surgery I tried almost every single remedy and product that others suggested. A few of these products didn't work but there were some that provided temporary relief.

Eventually, through a lot of trial and experimentation and researching for multiple hours a day, I found a winning formula that put me on the road to recovery.

Today I want to share this solution with you. I wish I'd had a resource (like the one I'm sharing with you now) or a knowledgeable person to turn to when I started my journey.

The information would have saved me from 6 months of hell.

Chapter 2

Differences Between Hemorrhoids & Fissures

Hemorrhoids are the result of pressure in the veins of the anus, which can arise from heavy lifting, giving birth or straining from a bowel movement.

This pressure causes the veins to bulge and expand.

Swollen, bulging veins are very painful, especially when sitting. Internal hemorrhoids are inside the anal opening. External hemorrhoids bulge out from the anal opening.

Usual symptoms of a hemorrhoid are:

- Anal itching
- Regular anal pain
- Bright red blood on the toilet paper
- Pain during bowel movements
- Hard tender lump near the anus

An anal fissure is the result of trauma to the inner lining of the anus. The fissure is literally a tear and occurs when a person has a tight anal sphincter muscle. It can also occur from frequent constipation or diarrhea.

The trauma causes the muscles in the anal sphincter to tear and this leads to a fissure. The tearing produces a lot of pain and causes the muscle to spasm.

When the anal sphincter muscle spasms, there is less blood flow to the site of the injury and this makes healing more difficult.

An anal fissure become chronic when the area cannot heal because of frequent spasm.

Usual symptoms of an anal fissure are:

- Severe pain during and after a bowel movement
- Bright red blood on the toilet paper and the stools

A key difference between an anal fissure and a hemorrhoid is that anal fissures are usually only painful during and after a bowel movement.

Hemorrhoids are painful throughout the day.

I'm guessing that you probably know what you have, but if you're like me then it's good to understand.

By looking at the list of symptoms above and identifying when the pain occurs, you can determine whether you have an anal fissure or a hemorrhoid.

Chapter 3

Common Causes Of An Anal Fissure

For some people it's not always obvious why an anal fissure develops. The most common reason is damage of the anal canal through a hard or painful bowel movement.

When this happens, the internal anal sphincter muscles tense up and spasm.

This reduces the blood supply to the area and makes it difficult for the tear to heal.

The issue is compounded by further hard bowel movements which can make the fissure come back or get worse.

Common reasons for developing an anal fissure are:

- Straining in a bowel movement due to constipation
- Pregnancy - because giving birth puts pressure on the perineum (in women this is the area between your anus and vulva)
- Inflammatory bowel disease, e.g. Crohn's Disease
- Sexually transmitted infection
- Psoriasis (dry, inflammatory skin)
- Opioid painkillers (side effects include constipation)
- Anal trauma through anal sex or hemorrhoid surgery
- Bowel cancer

Chapter 4

When I First Developed My Fissure

Aged 41, I was driving to a restaurant for a Christmas party and noticed an excruciating pain in my bottom. The pain felt unusual. I don't like taking medication unless I really need it.

But on this occasion, I had to take a painkiller. It eventually kicked in a couple of hours after I'd got to the party.

In the time that I was sitting down in the restaurant, waiting for my food order to arrive, the pain was excruciating.

All I could think about whilst browsing the menu was where the heck did this pain come from? I didn't have any other symptoms at the time.

As the days progressed, I started experiencing some pain when going to the bathroom in the mornings and every time I'd pass a bowel movement.

The pain would come and go and I didn't think much of it.

For the next 12 months, I noticed that if I ate more good fats in my diet (especially avocados), I could control my bowel movements and the pain in my anus would go away.

The days that I missed eating an avocado, I would experience a sharp anal pain the next morning after going to the bathroom.

Panic mode

I experienced my first blood loss with my bowel movements about 4 weeks after the Christmas party.

I think it's worth mentioning here that I lost my mother at a young age to bowel cancer.

I know that I have a gene that could trigger the same condition and that is why I started taking my health more seriously as soon as I hit 40.

I don't know the ins and outs of why my mother developed bowel cancer. I was too young at the time (a kid in school) to care much about my parents' health at the time.

As I grew older, I heard from other family members that her diet wasn't that great. She didn't consume much fiber and her exercise was limited.

My mother also had an office based job so she was sitting at a desk for long periods of time.

I remember as my mother got older (she died aged 51), she started putting on more weight.

A poor diet, lack of exercise and weight gain can all contribute towards a number of serious diseases.

Chapter 5

The Importance Of Diet For Healing A Fissure

For several years I've been eating a plant based vegetarian diet, which includes plenty of fiber, and I still got an anal fissure.

An anal fissure can occur because of hard stools and the resultant straining which causes a tear in the anal sphincter lining.

The pain from the tear comes about because of the large number of nerve endings in the anus.

It's really important that you drink plenty of water to aid your digestion and facilitate the movement of food through the intestine.

You need to drink a minimum of 2 quarts per day (yes ladies, that applies to you too!).

And if you're in hot weather then you should up this to 3 quarts or more.

(1 quart is just under 1 liter).

You also need to make sure that you're moving about enough.

If you lead a sedentary lifestyle (e.g. you sit a lot at a desk) then make sure you actively move several times a day by going for a 10 minute walk each time.

Here's my recommendations for your diet:

1. Cut out anything that's hard. This includes nuts, nut butters, highly chewy foods (e.g. processed meat), crusty bread, root vegetables like cassava, yam & plantain, hard cheeses and seeds.

2. Up your soft food intake. Ideally, this will include plenty of soups with vegetables (to get your fiber intake) and avoiding anything that won't take an age to digest like processed meat.

   I'm regularly on the go so I take soup in a thermal flask from home.

3. If you're not a big fan of green vegetables (like myself) then consider making green smoothies - they're really easy with a device like a Nutri Bullet, Nutri Ninja (https://amzn.to/2F3PSlf) or other similar type of blender.

   Don't make a smoothie with a traditional juicer. Instead you want a blender because it retains the fiber.

   I use several green vegetables and add a couple pieces of fruit so that the smoothie doesn't taste too bitter.

   I'm literally putting in a bowl's worth of chopped up green vegetables into the blender.

   The resultant mixture is really thick so I dilute the smoothie down with additional water to make it drinkable.

Is Your Doctor Wrong About Fiber?

Traditional medical advice for healing a fissure is to drink more water and up your fiber intake. This advice works if you're treating constipation or a mild/acute fissure.

But for chronic fissures (i.e. it's lasted longer than 6 weeks), upping your fiber intake with supplements like psyllium husk (Metamucil) could actually harm your recovery.

It sounds contradictory to what your Doctor might tell you but there's good reason for it.

When you're in the healing stage, you want to keep your stools small and soft. Natural fiber from fruits, vegetables and beans is fine.

But if you start adding in too much fiber, you'll bulk your stools and this can cause a re-tear.

The chart on the next page illustrates the pH levels of different foods. Most diets encourage the consumption of alkaline foods for optimal health.

If your food is mostly S.A.D. (standard American diet) then it's likely that you're consuming too much meat, dairy, bread, potatoes, sugar (desserts like ice cream and sugary soda beverages) and alcohol.

To rebalance your diet, consider upping your intake of fresh fruit and vegetables in an array of colours.

These will give you the nutrients that your body needs to keep you in good health.

The pH Of Food Chart

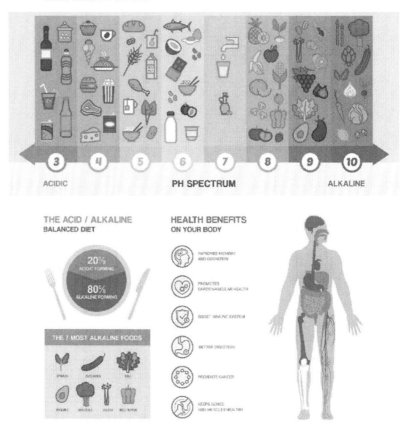

Healthier foods (fruits and vegetables) are on the right side of the chart.

Consuming more of these foods, whilst minimising consumption of foods on the left side of the chart, will give your body the nutrients that it needs to heal.

Chapter 6

Managing The Pain Of A Fissure

Priority ONE: Painkillers

The worst type of medications to use for fissure pain are the opioids - i.e. those with codeine, fentanyl, hydrocodone, meperidine, methadone, morphine, oxycodone.

These will make you constipated!

Stick to regular acetaminophen tablets (available from here: https://amzn.to/2XDPdyd) and ibuprofen tablets (available from here: https://amzn.to/2ItglE4).

You can use aspirin instead of ibuprofen but I prefer ibuprofen because it has stronger anti-inflammatory properties than regular aspirin.

You can safely take 2 acetaminophen 500mg tablets up to 4 times a day (i.e. every 4-6 hours apart).

In between you can use ibuprofen 400mg (or 2 x 200mg tablets) up to 3 times a day (or every 6-8 hours).

Whilst you can actually combine both pain relief medications, I recommend that you alternate them every 2 hours to get a continuous "drip feed" of pain relief.

Example Pain Relief Schedule

This schedule assumes that you're not on other pain relief medication. If you are, check with your Physician first.

- Adjust these times to suit you -

1) 7am: Take 2 x acetaminophen 500mg tablets.
2) 9am: Take 1 x ibuprofen 400mg tablet.
3) 11am: Take 2 x acetaminophen 500mg tablets.
4) 1pm: Take 1 x ibuprofen 400mg tablet.
5) 3pm: Take 2 x acetaminophen 500mg tablets.
6) 5pm: Take 1 x ibuprofen 400mg tablet.
7) 7pm: Take 2 x acetaminophen 500mg tablets.

This should carry you through to around 9-10pm (close to bed time) for pain relief.

With ibuprofen, you need to take this with or after food. So, if you're eating 3 meals a day, take an ibuprofen 400mg with each meal.

If you're still in agony come 9pm, you can take a 4th ibuprofen 400mg tablet for the day.

It's not recommended to take more than 3 x 400mg ibuprofen tablets per day but in the short term, my Physician told me that it's fine to increase to a 4th ibuprofen tablet.

I recommend that you consult with your own Physician to best manage your pain.

Personally, I found that I'd get the maximum benefit from a painkiller approximately 2 hours after taking it.

Remember, blood flow to the anus is restricted when you have a fissure, so it's logical that pain relief will take longer to kick in than it would for other types of pain like a headache.

So, if you know that you're going to be regular for a bowel movement at around 9am, take a painkiller about 7am.

If you forget to wake up earlier, you can use soluble pain relief tablets. Dissolving a tablet in water gets it into the blood stream faster.

I would always be in maximum pain shortly after having a bowel movement. The pain would progressively get worse for several hours.

If this is happening to you, it's because the secondary anal sphincter muscle is going into spasm.

The spasm restricts the blood supply. When the anal sphincter muscle spasms, it also contracts and this causes sharp pain.

Priority TWO: Stool Softeners

You MUST (and I cannot emphasise this enough) keep your stools soft. If your stools remain hard, it will be impossible for your fissure to heal because you'll keep on tearing it regularly.

Aim for a consistency of between 3 to 5 for your stools. At levels 1 and 2 you are constipated and this means more painful bowel movements.

Poop Chart

chart of poop

	1. Very hard lungs separated
	2. Compact but lumpy
	3. Soft like a sausage with cracks
	4. Like a sausage but soft
	5. Whit soft balls
	6. Very soft with jagged edges
	7. Entirely liquid

I used Docusate Sodium capsules to help me get a softer consistency: 2 capsules with a heavy meal or 1 capsule with a light meal.

You can safely take 5 capsules in a day.

Brand names for Docusate Sodium are Dioctyl & DulcoEase.

Get it here: https://amzn.to/2MFt9ly

Softer stools also mean less pain when you have a bowel movement.

Moderate exercise that gets your heart rate up e.g. walking/running/ swimming, getting enough fiber (don't over-do it with medication) and drinking enough water will also help you to pass soft, regular stools.

If you're a gym bunny (like me) you should avoid lifting heavy weights. Straining can cause a re-tear of a fissure. If you're worried about losing muscle tone, use a lighter weight and increase the reps.

Some upper body exercises like dumb bell curls, pull ups and lat pull-downs are fine, but you definitely want to avoid lower body exercises like squats, lunges and deadlifts.

If you want to speed up your healing process, I recommend that you exercise daily. Even a short 5-10 minute run will help to encourage blood flow all around the body.

If you can't manage a run because of physical health problems then do your best to get in a brisk walk every day or a swim.

Having a sedentary lifestyle probably contributed to you getting an anal fissure.

Maintaining a sedentary lifestyle won't help you to heal.

Priority THREE: Quality Toilet Paper

Now is not the time to skimp on the quality of your toilet paper. You must go for the softest type that you can afford.

Here is a soft, quilted toilet paper that I recommend for you: https://amzn.to/2XDukmF

If you're stuck at work/need to use a public restroom and have to rely on inferior quality toilet paper, make sure that you're able to clean yourself thoroughly.

Your fissure is an open wound and even the smallest amount of soil, left-over from your stools, will leave you in agony.

Here's a quick tip: don't aggressively wipe with dry toilet paper. Doing so could damage the skin in the anal canal (where it's already sensitive) and increase your pain.

Instead, wet the toilet paper to clean more efficiently and then use wet wipes after if needed.

I recommend these wet wipes: https://amzn.to/2Wx21Fh as they have lidocaine which is a numbing agent. Lidocaine will help with the pain.

Some wipes block the toilet pipes so don't flush the wipes! You can safely dispose of them by using a diaper sack. Available here: https://amzn.to/2H7hiYy

I'd also recommend that at the end of your cleaning session, you get some additional toilet roll and dab it in some coconut oil.

Then wipe your bottom with it. I use this coconut oil: https://amzn.to/2X6naub

This will help to clean the area and remove any left-over soil.

Additionally, you can dab some colloidal silver inside your anal cheeks. Available here: https://amzn.to/2IyJNOx

I found that colloidal silver, combined with the coconut oil, helped to reduce my post bowel movement pain. Both these products have anti-bacterial properties.

A good way to reduce the discomfort from a spasm, after a bowel movement, is to use a sitz bath.

Sitz bath kit available here: https://amzn.to/2Wx0f75

Sitz bath soaks available here: https://amzn.to/2MAKPyH

If a sitz bath isn't practical for you, try purchasing a detachable shower head (with hose) to use at home on your bottom.

You can purchase these at most hardware shops or from Amazon: https://amzn.to/2YXKdEr

Simply attach the shower hose to a bathroom faucet and rinse thoroughly inside your anal cheeks with warm or hot water.

Chapter 7

Treating Your Fissure

Disclaimer: not every treatment that worked/didn't work for me will have the same results for you because our bodies respond differently.

The products listed are ones that I used to recover and that also helped others. Appropriate use of all the recommended products will improve the rate at which you heal.

You need to be realistic about the healing process: a chronic fissure can take weeks or even months to heal.

The anus doesn't receive as much blood supply as other parts of the body which means that the healing process is longer than for an ordinary cut.

To give your body the best chance to heal, you need to improve your immune system. This means eating healthy and taking supplements.

If you've skipped Chapter 5 (The Importance Of Diet For Healing A Fissure) please go back and read it now. It's really important that you choose your food carefully!

If you don't control the size and bulk of your stools (which all depends on what you eat) then you're going to struggle each time you have a bowel movement and cause a re-tear.

Aim for 1-2 bowel movements per day. Staying regular will help to keep your stools small.

If you leave it more than 24 hours in between bowel movements the stool will get bigger. You want to avoid this because a bigger stool will increase the risk of a re-tear.

If you're struggling to have a bowel movement at least once a day, speak to your Physician about using laxatives.

Note: links to all of the recommended products in this book can be found at: https://www.healanalfissure.com/products

Treatments That Did Not Work (For Me)

1. *Rectiv ™ Ointment* (nitroglycerin) is available over the counter in Australia under the brand name Rectogesic™ but in most countries is prescribed by a medical Doctor. A common side effect is headache.

   The manufacturer recommends using Rectiv ™ twice a day but I suffered really bad headaches from it and could only use it at bed time.

   Rectiv ™ works by increasing the blood flow to the fissure area.

   I tried Rectiv ™ for 2 weeks before giving up because of the side effects. I didn't notice any improvement in those 2 weeks.

2. *Organic Turmeric* – it's good for arthritic pains but turmeric didn't help in healing my fissure.

3. *Hemosan Cream* - this made my post bowel itching even worse. Instead of cooling the anal area, it created a burning sensation.

4. *Himalaya Herbas Pilex* tablets/ointment -> the tablets didn't do anything. The ointment gave some light relief as a barrier but didn't improve my fissure.

5. *Frankincense Oil* - it's helped others but I didn't notice any difference.

6. *Ma Ying Long Musk Hemorrhoids Ointment* - like Hemosan, this made the burning sensation worse.

Treatments That Helped Me Recover & That I Recommend For You

1. **Dulcolax** - to soften your stools (contains gelatine).
Available from: https://amzn.to/2MFt9ly

2. **Miralax** (gelatine free stool softener).
Available from: https://amzn.to/2IgcHeq

3. **Metamucil Fiber** - helps to keep your stools regular.
Available from: https://amzn.to/2WCH7cD

- You only need Metamucil if your diet lacks fiber. Ideally, you should get your fiber by consuming fresh fruit and vegetables on a regular basis.

4. **Tylenol (Acetaminophen)** - for effective pain relief.
Available from: https://amzn.to/2XDPdyd

5. **Advil (Ibuprofen)** - for effective pain relief. Is also an anti-inflammatory.
Available from: https://amzn.to/2ItgIE4

6. **Quilted Toilet Roll** - for a softer wipe post bowel movement. Get it here: https://amzn.to/2XDukmF

7. **Magnesium Citrate (Pure Encapsulations)** - anti-inflammatory & helps keeps your stools regular. Available from: https://amzn.to/2WxIPvM

8. **Vitamin C Tablets** - a strong antioxidant to boost your immune system.
Available from: https://amzn.to/2XDbqwb

9. **H-Fissure Oil** - A natural cure that contains homeopathic ingredients. Use a cotton swab to apply the oil directly onto the fissure 2-3 times a day.

   I purchased the larger 33ml size bottle and noticed a big improvement to my fissure within a few weeks. Available from: https://tinyurl.com/h-fissures-oil

10. **Doctor Butler's Hemorrhoid & Fissure Ointment** - helps to soothe the anus from burning and itching. Available from: https://amzn.to/2KCc7Cq

11. **Recticare Cream** - helps to soothe the anus from burning, pain and itching.
Available from: https://amzn.to/2IDi0g9

12. **Recticare Wipes** - to help clean the anus thoroughly after a bowel movement.
Available from: https://amzn.to/2Wx21Fh

13. **Ano-Sitz Bath Kit** - to help with the pain from muscular spasms post bowel movement.
Available from: https://amzn.to/2Wx0f75

14. **Sitz Bath Soaks** - to help with the pain from muscular spasms after a bowel movement.
Available from: https://amzn.to/2MAKPyH

15. **Organic H Salve** - to help soothe the anus from burning/itching.
Available from: https://amzn.to/2F0CtKQ

16. **Aloe Vera Gel** - cools the anus and reduces burning.
Available from: https://amzn.to/31tVA9N

17. **Colloidal Silver Cream** - an antibacterial to relieve sting and help aid recovery.
Available from: https://amzn.to/2IyJNOx

18. **Vita Virgin Coconut Oil** - helps to clean and soothe post bowel movement.
Available from: https://amzn.to/2X6naub

19. **Shea Butter Organic** - soothes and aids recovery.
Available from: https://amzn.to/2WFHeUX

20. **Probiotics 60 Billion** - to help aid recovery and boost your immune system.
Available from: https://amzn.to/2WvldmL

21. **Zinc (Pure Encapsulations)** - to help heal cuts and boost your immune system.
Available from: https://amzn.to/2IBYaBD

22. **Vaseline** - as a lubricant to help bowel movements (use before and after).
Available from: https://amzn.to/2MBwlPc

23. **Nutri Ninja** - for blending foods to make them easier to consume. I use it for making green smoothies. Available from: https://amzn.to/2F3PSlf

24. **Wheatgrass Powder** - helps to keep your stools soft. I use it in my green smoothies. Available from: https://amzn.to/2JTsBnx

25. **Desitin Zinc Cream** - promotes healing of the fissure (the cream is fine to use with zinc tablets). Available from: https://amzn.to/2YfpXBJ

26. **Calmoseptine Cream** – relief of burning and itching. Available from: https://amzn.to/2Sx4yPI

27. **Uriage Barrier Ointment** - helps to heal the fissure by forming a protective barrier. Make sure you get it high enough into the anal canal to cover the fissure. Available from: https://amzn.to/2Y5EnR5

Tip: crouch on the floor with a mirror under you to identify where the fissure is. Take a new cotton swab and use it to apply the ointment.

If you're in a lot of pain, take a painkiller first and wait for it to kick in before using the cotton swab.

Chapter 8

Alternative Therapies: Kegel Exercises & Massage

Kegel Exercises

Also known as pelvic floor exercises. You can do these on your own and at any time by contracting and releasing the sphincter muscle (the one you use to stop urine flow).

Practice holding the muscle for 3 seconds and then releasing several times a day. The main benefit is that you'll strengthen the sphincter muscle.

Note: If you're a female and have a weak pelvic floor (e.g. after giving birth) then consult with your Physician first to determine the right type of exercise for you.

Here is a resource that you can visit for more information before you see your Physician:

https://torontophysiotherapy.ca/do-kegels-work-are-kegels-bad-for-you

Gluteal Massages

Having a gluteal massage, whether it's from a professional masseuse or a healthcare professional like a chiropractor or osteopath can bring huge relief to the pain of an anal fissure and encourage healing.

Gluteal massages stimulate the flow of blood into the anus, where it's already restricted.

Ask for help from a partner, a family member or a friend if receiving regular massages from a professional isn't practical.

A daily gluteal massage will speed up your recovery time.

Chapter 9

Coping At Work And Your Social Life

Dealing With Social Issues

If you have people in your life that you trust, please don't isolate yourself.

Right now, you need the help and emotional support of your family and close friends. You'll feel better if you open up about your condition.

Talking through issues will help you to stay positive.

Your close friends, and the ones that are worth keeping, will understand why there might be times when you can't socialise or eat and drink with them.

1-1 Consultation Support

I understand that getting help, support or advice from family and friends is not always practical, or even possible, so for a limited time I am offering you the opportunity to have a 1-1 consultation with me.

This consultation is for you if you're too embarrassed to approach family or friends.

It's also for you if you'd prefer to speak to someone that understands what you're going through and who can personally guide you on your road to recovery.

Note: I reserve the right to remove this offer for 1-1 support because there's only one of me.

If you've got questions and don't know where to turn, or if you're looking to speed up the recovery from your anal fissure, you should schedule an appointment right **now**.

Visit: https://www.healanalfissure.com/consultation for more information.

Why We Need Oxytocin To Heal

When we stay connected to our close family and friends, a hormone called oxytocin is released in our body.

Oxytocin is produced in the hypothalamus part of the brain. It's commonly referred to as the 'love hormone' because it helps promote feelings of love, bonding and well-being.

Scientific studies have shown that oxytocin helps with wound healing. It plays a key role in 'angiogenesis', which is the growth of blood vessels or re-growth of them after an injury.

Research shows that wounds take longer to heal when people are under stress or are involved in an emotional conflict. These people have lower oxytocin levels.

Even if you've had an anal fissure for a long time (some people live with the condition for years), don't give up hope.

You can still recover by following the steps in this book. Remind yourself that your situation is temporary and not permanent.

As you start to heal your life will improve. And if you manage your pain relief effectively then it's still possible to have a social life.

Dealing With Work

Coping at work with an anal fissure can be a tricky situation. If you're in a shared office space, then you'll likely be sharing the restrooms too.

Ideally, you'd have access to a private cubicle with its own sink in the restroom but I know this isn't possible for everyone.

I learned to cope by training my body to have an early morning bowel movement.

This gave me an opportunity to use the bathroom at home in a familiar and relaxed environment. I'm sure most people would prefer to use their own bathroom instead of a public restroom.

At home you have an opportunity to clean yourself thoroughly and jump into the shower or use a sitz bath after a bowel movement.

In a public restroom that opportunity becomes more challenging.

Here's a few tips that may help:

1. Diet

Start by consuming extra fiber with your evening meal the night before you go to work. If you're eating out, take Metamucil with plenty of water.

Metamucil available here: https://amzn.to/2WCH7cD

On the actual day of work, wake up 30 minutes earlier than normal and have a hot drink: it doesn't matter whether it's tea, coffee or hot water with lemon.

The hot drink will help to facilitate a bowel movement.

And if it doesn't, try combining the hot drink with breakfast.

Most of us experience a bowel movement after breakfast.

2. Laxatives

If you're still struggling to get a morning bowel movement at home through your diet, consider using a laxative like Lactulose or Miralax the night before.

Miralax available here: https://amzn.to/2lgcHeq

This will help you get into a routine. I recommend that you speak to your Physician first though.

3. Eat Regularly

When you're at work try to resist long breaks in between meals.

You'll end up stuffing yourself with extra food because of the hunger pangs and this will make your stools bulkier.

Drink a full glass of water before your meals. Our bodies often confuse hunger with thirst.

Also, chew your food more slowly. It takes 20 minutes for the stomach to signal to the brain that it's eaten enough food.

4. Stool Softeners

I recommend that you keep a small amount of Dioctyl with you at all times.

Dioctyl available here: https://amzn.to/2MFt9ly

This way you're always covered for stool softeners, whether you're having lunch at work or eating out with colleagues or friends.

If you haven't got a small container to put the Dioctyl capsules in, ask in a local Pharmacy for a tablet bottle that you can keep in your pocket or bag.

You can also use sachets of Miralax powder instead of Dioctyl capsules.

Miralax powder available here: https://amzn.to/2TrAghv

5. Chair Support

Some people use a donut shaped seat cushion to put on their work chair.

Donut cushion available here: https://amzn.to/2YyDjsV

These cushions help to relieve pain in the tailbone and coccyx (lower back) area. They're also useful for relief of pain from hemorrhoids and fissures.

If you're going to use one of these cushions, don't sit on it for too long. You'll end up applying prolonged pressure to your fissure which could make it more painful after.

6. Wet Wipes

There will be times when you need to use a public or work restroom. The most effective way to clean yourself in public is with wet wipes.

Wet wipes are more convenient and discrete than using a portable sitz bath kit.

Recticare wipes contain glycerin and lidocaine to soothe and help with the itching. They also provide pain relief.

Available here: https://amzn.to/2Wx21Fh

Chapter 10

Coping With Stress: Developing A Positive Attitude

Mindset & Stress

Henry Ford, world famous business leader and founder of the Ford Motor Company, once said: "Whether you think you can or whether you think you can't, you're right."

Our mind has remarkable powers to heal the body. Our thoughts, feelings and expectations have a profound influence on our well-being.

It's widely known that having a positive outlook will help to ease physical pain.

On the flip side, enduring long term stress and negativity in our lives can have an adverse reaction on our health.

You don't need to be a Physician to understand that stress can impact your body in so many ways: it can trigger tension headaches, cause depression and make it difficult to sleep.

Stress also plays havoc with your hormones; leaving you with a weakened immune system and high blood pressure.

So, what's the solution?

The answer is to reduce stress and negativity in your life.

Perhaps you have a difficult job with long hours or you have problems in a relationship with a family member, your spouse or a business partner?

Negative energies can impact your body in so many ways.

The longer you let these negative energies manifest, the more problems they will cause in your life.

You need to evaluate what is important to you and what is worth letting go. When you find the balance between positive and negative energy, you'll find peace.

On a scientific level, it's already been proven that people with stress and emotional conflict, e.g. those who are in a difficult relationship, have lower levels of oxytocin.

(Oxytocin is responsible for wound healing. Read Chapter 9 for more on this.)

I'm not here to get deeply spiritual or "woo-woo" on you. But I do believe that energy forces exist in nature and so I'll share what I tried and what helped me.

When I had an anal fissure, I was desperate to heal and willing to try almost anything, within reason and the boundaries of the law, to get back to normality.

Relaxation & How To Balance Your Life Force Energies (Chakras)

Before we get into this, I encourage you to suspend any limiting beliefs and give this a go. Remember what Henry Ford said? Whatever you believe in, you're right.

I recommend you try the following: you've got little to lose and much to potentially gain.

Agreed? Ok here goes:

1. **Spend Time In Nature**

   Even if you live in a big city (like I do), go to a local park and start walking barefoot on the grass. Touch a tree, be near a waterfall, engage with wildlife (birds, ducks, deer etc.) and feel the sun on you.

2. **Practice Creative Visualization**

   Clear your mind and think happy thoughts. Picture a flower opening or the bliss that you felt when you met a loved one.

3. **Breathe Deeply**

   Doing this will instantly lower your blood pressure. Take a deep breath in and then slowly exhale. Repeat several times and you'll start to relax.

4. **Start Journaling**

   Just the act of writing down what happened to you (both positive and negative) during the day can help to release stress from your body. It's up to you if you wish to keep your records or destroy them after.

5. **Practice Gratitude**

   You don't have to wait for Thanksgiving for this. Be grateful for what you have in your life and say it out loud.

You can practice gratitude by taking a minute every day, e.g. when you're getting ready in the morning, on your commute to work or before you go to bed at night.

If you want to go deeper on this topic here's an article on Deepak Chopra's site:

https://chopra.com/articles/how-to-balance-your-chakras-without-reiki

In case you've not heard of him, Deepak Chopra is an American-Indian Doctor that is famous for alternative medicine and spiritual thinking.

Chapter 11

Meditation

Modern science is finally recognizing the benefits of meditation in our busy, stressful lives.

You don't need to go to extremes and become a practising yogi to benefit. Even 5 minutes a day can give you results.

Benefits Of Meditation

1. Relaxation

We learn to relax in a deep way by calming our minds. This puts us into a state of deep physiological rest.

Consider how refreshed you feel in the morning after a good night's sleep. Meditation re-energises our mind.

Our bodies maintain balance through homeostasis. When the body is in balance it's able to prevent illness and to heal.

Meditation restores the body's natural balance, physically and emotionally.

2. Improved Decision Making

By calming our minds, we obtain clarity of thought. Think about the times when you've had a creative idea pop into your head: were you relaxed or stressed?

Many people find solutions to their problems when they're in the bath/shower or when they're relaxing in bed as they drift off to sleep.

Our mind decides what we're going to eat, how we're going to behave with others, whether we exercise, what we drink and what sort of treatments we'll have.

Meditation allows us to think clearly, make better decisions and commit to following through. An example is a decision to exercise daily to become healthier and speed up recovery.

3. Be More Authentic

On a spiritual level (whatever your beliefs), meditation will help you feel more connected.

Even if you're not religious you can choose nature or the Universe as your source to feel connected and confident.

4. Guided Imagery

Using mind-body medicine we can promote healing with our minds. Guided imagery works on the principle that thoughts which pass through our mind create internal images.

To the body and nervous system these thoughts are indistinguishable from actual physical reality.

By creating a positive inner image (of your body, health or performance) we can use our subconscious mind to promote healing and make our thoughts a reality.

Guided imagery is not just for healing: many top athletes in the world use visualization to enhance their performance.

5. State Of Mind

We can influence how we feel by focusing on the positives or the negatives in every situation.

An example is the question: "is the glass half full or half empty?". How you answer this proverbial phrase defines your view of the world. Are you an optimist or a pessimist?

Meditation lets our mind gravitate towards healing qualities. We find it easy to be joyful when our mind is rested and at peace.

When we are rested a natural optimism comes out and we find it easy to laugh. Laughter really is **'the best medicine'**.

It improves our state of mind and has a positive influence on our health.

6. Reduce Stress

Stress is a major cause of inflammation in our body and can manifest in different ways, e.g. tight chest pains, tension headaches or an upset stomach.

Prolonged inflammation leads to disease.

Meditation helps by regulating the stress response.

When we are relaxed, our gut bacteria release short chain fatty acids that provide anti-inflammatory and anti-tumor effects.

If you'd like to find out more about meditation, a great resource is Deepak Chopra's site: https://chopra.com

How Meditation Helped Me To Heal

The premise of this book is to give you the same actionable steps that I used to heal my fissure, so in this section I'm going to share what worked for me.

Other sufferers of anal fissures recommended a couple of short mantras to me and now I'd like to share them so that you too can benefit.

You don't have to be religious to believe that there are energy forces in nature.

These forces are powerful enough to make us fall ill if we have an imbalance in our chakra energies. But if we work towards balancing these forces, we can help ourselves to heal and stay healthy.

The mantra videos that helped me are only a few minutes long and I recommend that you watch both. I felt relaxed and at peace watching them. I hope you experience the same.

Copy the URLs into your browser (or search in YouTube ™) to watch the videos.

Mantra 1: Medicine Buddha Mantra.

Tayata Om Bekandze

Bekandze Maha Bekandze

Randze Samud Gate Soha

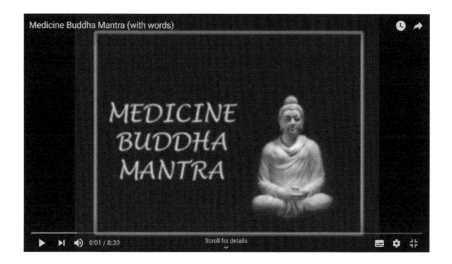

Available here: https://youtu.be/yUJucA-mrgE

Translation:

May the sentient beings who are sick, quickly be freed from sickness.

And may all the sicknesses of beings never arise again.

Meaning:

'Bekandze' means eliminating pain.

'Maha Bekandze' means great elimination of pain.

The first 'Bekandze' refers to eliminating the pain of suffering, not just of disease but of all problems.

The second 'Bekandze' eliminates the cause of suffering that arises from karma and disturbing thoughts.

Mantra 2: Tina Turner - Peace Mantra

Sarveśām Svastir Bhavatu

Sarveśām Shāntir Bhavatu

Sarveśām Pūrnam Bhavatu

Sarveśām Maṇgalam Bhavatu

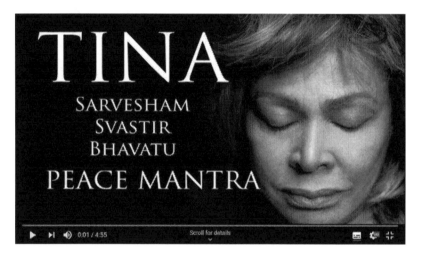

Available here: https://youtu.be/6XP-f7wPM0A

Translation:

May there be happiness in all.

May there be peace in all.

May there be completeness in all.

May there be success in all.

Meaning:

'Sarvesham' - all, everything

'Svastir' - health, well-being

'Bhavatu' - may there be

'Shanti' - peace

'Pūrnam' - completeness, fulfilment

'Mangalam' - spiritual success, prosperity

Chapter 12

Traditional Medical Treatments For A Fissure

If you have tried all of the above treatments and they haven't helped your anal fissure to heal, you may have a more serious condition that requires surgery.

Ask your Physician to refer you to a Colorectal Surgeon (CRS). You may want to seek the opinion of more than one.

The surgeon will discuss options for treating your anal fissure. Some of these may include:

1. Botox (Botulinum Toxin) Injections

Here the surgeon applies the injection directly into your internal sphincter muscle. The aim is to temporarily relax this muscle so that your fissure can heal.

2. Fissurectomy

This involves cutting away the damaged skin from around your anal fissure, along with any skin tags (lumps of skin associated with the fissure) that have developed.

Your surgeon may suggest that you have this alongside Botox injections.

3. Lateral Internal Sphincterotomy

This type of surgery is considered 'the gold standard' for treating anal fissures.

The surgery involves cutting the lower part of the internal sphincter muscle around the anus to relieve the spasm in the sphincter.

Stopping the spasm restores blood supply to the area and gives the fissure a chance to heal.

4. Anal Advancement Flaps

This procedure involves taking healthy skin from your anal lining and using it to replace the broken skin in your fissure.

You can have it at the same time as a sphincterotomy or afterwards if your fissure doesn't heal.

Positives Of Surgery

Most patients make a quick recovery and can return home on the same day after surgery.

The pain from a fissure will rapidly improve. Some people can return back to work within a few days of the surgery, depending on the physical nature of their work.

With regular exercise (to improve blood circulation) you can quickly resume normal activity.

Negatives Of Surgery

Irrespective of which option you choose, there is still a possibility of the fissure returning.

And this likelihood increases if you repeat the circumstances that led to the fissure in the first place, e.g. lack of exercise, poor diet, constipation.

General complications of surgery include:

- Pain
- Bleeding
- Infection at the wound site

Specific complications of surgery include:

- Involuntarily passing wind or loose bowel movements from lost control
- Difficulty passing urine
- Permanent incontinence from the bowel

If you are seriously thinking about surgery, don't just seek the opinion of your nearest Colorectal Surgeon. It can be worth traveling to a different state.

Also do your homework: ask your Physician and any other healthcare professionals in your network (friends/family) for referrals.

You may also want to consider using LinkedIn ™ to find a top Colorectal Surgeon.

Chapter 13

My Personal Thoughts On Surgery

I confess that I have an irrational fear when it comes to hospitals and medical procedures.

Perhaps it's distrust through reading one too many horror stories in the media about a botched operation.

Or maybe it's the over exposure to hospitals that I had from a young age: I was still a kid in school when I lost my mother to bowel cancer.

It was a traumatic experience to visit her in the hospital and see her deteriorating in the hospital bed, waiting months for the inevitable cruel end.

More recently, when I suffered with an anal fissure, I used to dread going to the bathroom. After having a bowel movement all I could think of was the pain.

And I was desperate for the pain to end.

Sometimes, the thought of surgery would flash through my head but I just couldn't pluck up the courage to ask my Physician for a referral.

Not after I'd researched the risks of surgery: how the fissure can recur and the risk of suffering involuntary fecal incontinence.

I'm sure there are success stories of people who've had surgery for an anal fissure and that have gone on to make a full recovery. The problem is tracking them down!

When people make a recovery, they go back to their normal, busy lives as they no longer have a need to participate in group chats.

It's human nature and most of us are guilty of it.

Think about the last time you had a fabulous experience at a restaurant.

Did you stop to leave a review on the Internet for the restaurant so that others could benefit from the experience?

Or do you only leave reviews when the experience is bad?

Surgery can be a quick fix and if you have the resources and a trusted surgeon to turn to then this might be a better option for you.

Personally, I wanted to try the non-invasive route and only use surgery as a last resort if all other methods failed, i.e. through diet, lifestyle and using the right medications.

But my healing didn't miraculously happen overnight.

It happened by changing my thoughts, changing my lifestyle and combining all the methods that I've laid out in this book.

Only then did I slowly start to heal my chronic anal fissure.

If you have patience and a positive attitude then it's possible that you can start the healing process without needing surgery.

If you're giving serious consideration to surgery then I invite you to arrange a 1-1 consultation with me before you commit.

Visit: https://www.healanalfissure.com/consultation for more information.

But, if you're looking for the quick option and you've exhausted all other methods then surgery may be your last resort.

Chapter 14

Additional Support From The Author

Having an anal fissure can be a lonely process.

Your family, friends and work colleagues may never understand what you're going through until they experience it for themselves.

For that reason, I've put together a package where you can receive on-going support, via email, from me for a full 30 days.

There is a cost to this but it's a small price to shortcut your suffering.

(I wish I'd had this support when I was in hell with my fissure.)

For the cost of a daily Starbucks ™ you'll receive an email every day over the next month that is packed with practical advice and tips.

You'll get in depth information on top of what I could fit into this book.

But it goes beyond just information…

I recently discovered a shocking fact:

Did you know that only 6% of medical graduates in the U.S. receive any formal training on nutrition?

What we eat has a huge impact on our health and our body's ability to recover from disease.

If you've been to see your Physician and only been told about traditional medical procedures, instead of being given nutritional advice to improve your health, now you know why.

I have recently invested hundreds of hours into learning as much as I can about nutrition, spiritual therapy and how to stay healthy.

And now I want to distil this knowledge and leave you with a plan that shows you how to overhaul your lifestyle and become a healthier version of yourself.

Over the next 30 days I'll share my journey with you and support you on your road to recovery.

Imagine what life would be like if you no longer had to fear going to the bathroom or using a public restroom?

Imagine how returning to normal life would feel:

- without experiencing pain from a bowel movement

- without having to roll around in discomfort for hours after?

In the next 30 days I'll show you how to heal your fissure naturally and how to stop it from recurring.

There's no fluff in these emails, it's simply actionable advice from my own hellish experience that you can use in your path to recovery.

Yes, I Want 30 Days Of Email Support
From Sam Summers

Visit this page to get started:

https://www.HealAnalFissure.com/support

Chapter 15

Review Request/Feedback

Thank you for reading this book. I sincerely hope that it's helped to improve your health and put you on the road to recovery.

I would appreciate if you could spare a few minutes to leave a review on Amazon at:

https://www.amazon.com/Healing-Anal-Fissure-Permanently-Resorting-ebook/dp/B07XKDSQ7M

(Short link: https://tinyurl.com/heal-fissure)

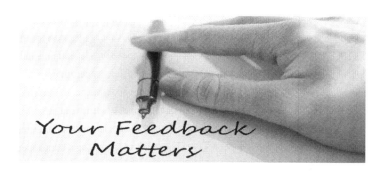

Your feedback will help others to benefit from the methods that I've shared.

If this book did not meet your expectations can you help me to improve it?

My mission is to help other people suffering from this awful condition and give them hope for a recovery.

A personal review or feedback from you can make a big difference in reaching someone that needs the information in this book.

If your feedback has value to others, I'll be happy to share it (with your permission) and give you credit on the website:

https://www.healanalfissure.com

And, if you've managed to cure your anal fissure - whether it's through the methods that I've explained in this book or in a different way - I would also love to hear your success story.

You can reach me here: support@HealAnalFissure.com

Thank you & good luck in your recovery!

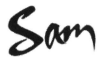

Sam Summers

Printed in Great Britain
by Amazon

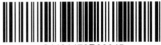

34401476R00045